I0429117

Swimming for Babies

7 Reasons why swimming is good for your baby

Mark Dube

Swimming for Babies
7 Reasons why swimming is good for your baby

ISBN-13: 978-1500633394
ISBN-10: 1500633399

Swimming is a life saving skill, as well as a holistic and simple exercise with benefits that go beyond physical development and improved health. Swimming stimulates intelligence and extends lifespan. Swimming can prevent your child from drowning, which is a major cause of death in young children. Swimming is fun and imparts long-lasting happiness. This book explains highly effective methods and strategies to teach babies the art of swimming at an early age. It also explains all the associated preparations, precautions as well as benefits that your child will reap on learning to swim. You will learn all the aspects of baby swimming from this book like:

- Benefits of swimming
- Reasons to start early Influence of parent on baby swimming
- Preparations, precautions, hygiene and safety during baby swimming
- Proven strategies to teach babies to swim from infant stage to six years

SWIMMING FOR BABIES

CONTENTS

SWIMMING FOR BABIES

1. BABIES CAN SWIM

A look at any baby instantly tickles our cuteness senses. We feel that the baby is beautiful, immovable and weak, therefore, is in need of protection. In-fact, a thought, never crosses our mind that he could be an expert swimmer! A newborn infant would have already been swimming for almost seven months in his mother's womb. Every newborn is an expert swimmer!

Let me explain.

During the first three weeks of pregnancy, your baby is just a rapidly growing ball of multiplying cells. At four weeks, the baby grows up to the size of a poppy seed. This marks the initiation of formation and development of all the organs. Six weeks from here, the baby will have all the organs formed. Off-course, very tiny to be distinguished even using medical devices. During 6 to seven weeks, heart starts beating and limbs bud out. At eight weeks, the arms, legs and fingers develop. Weighing 400th of an ounce and measuring just 5/8th of an inch, he starts moving rapidly with his newly formed limbs.

His mother does not feel it as he is very tiny. He is swimming and exploring the fluidly filled womb of his mother. By four months, his arms and legs are large enough to be felt by his mother. He will start kicking harder from here, often waking his mother from sleep. He cares no more; he is just enjoying the swim.

Every newborn is a trained swimmer with 7 months of practice. He is an expert at swimming in the womb. With a bit of training, he can learn quickly to swim in the pool as well. In the womb, he was swimming without a purpose. In the real world, swimming will be a very big advantage. It could even save his life someday.

Babies can swim well before they can crawl, creep or walk. The floor is a completely different playground to fluidly filled womb in which babies grow and swim during pregnancy. The newborns know the feel of the fluid but not the floor. With a little practice, the newborns can learn to swim in the pool without any assistance. On the contrary, they will lose their swimming abilities if they are not trained consistently. This is the reason many baby-swimming schools insist on coaching babies from a very early age. Some of them even suggest starting to teach the baby from the first day of birth.

Age is the biggest enemy for learning to swim. With every passing day, swimming learning abilities decline. It is easier to teach a 4-year-old to swim than a 5-year-old or a 1-year-old than a 4-year-old. In the case of newborns, there is even no need of teaching them how to swim because they already know. This is only the opportunity to use their skills acquired in the womb in the real world.

The benefits of teaching babies to swim are many and significant. Read on this in the next section.

SWIMMING FOR BABIES

2. BENEFITS OF LEARNING TO SWIM EARLY

The thoughts that come into our minds when considering swimming are its health promoting and life saving potentials. Most of us learn to swim as a lifesaving skill. Learning to swim is a simple yet powerful way to acquire plenty of benefits especially for babies. They will go on to live a better life with these benefits. Let us have a look at scientifically documented benefits of swimming from early childhood. This list is not exhaustive. You are free to grow it with other benefits you know of or have experienced.

A. It is the best way to learn water safety

National Center for Injury Prevention and Control, a constituent body of Centers for Disease Control and Prevention, reported that drowning is the third leading cause of unintentional injury or death worldwide. This accounts for more than 359,000 deaths (7% of all injury-related deaths) every year worldwide. The World Health Organisation (WHO) believes that these facts are likely to be overly underestimated. Unfortunately, more than 20% of the deaths are among children aged less than 14 years. Furthermore, drowning is the second major cause of death after congenital anomalies/deformities (birth defects) among children aged 1 to four years old. Drowning can occur under various circumstances; however, the inability to swim remains the major cause of drowning.

Why are we losing plenty of babies to drowning? This could easily be prevented through early swimming coaching. In addition to the swimming skills there are other techniques which are learnt while swimming. Such techniques include the ability to hold under water, the ability to get out of water or the ability to swim to the side that can save life one day.

An example of 2-year-old Elizabeth Jelley, from Wirral, United Kingdom, who fell into the family pool. She was sure to drown to death; luckily, she had started learning to swim from 7 weeks of age. This helped her to come to the surface, swim to the side and hold on for over eight minutes leading her mother to find her.

B. Best exercise out there to gain physical and mental health!

No other exercise packs the health benefits that your baby can reap from swimming from early childhood. In addition to health, the baby will develop a keen interest in sports. This keenness could last a lifetime. Every stroke of a swim provides a complete workout for the muscles, lungs, heart and most importantly the brain. In turn, all the 5 pillars of human sensations: sound, sight, smell, touch and taste are stimulated. Here is an outline of ten scientifically proven benefits.

a. *More gain with the least effort:* Swimming is the least stressful exercise compared to any other workout that can yield reward similar benefits to the body. Swimming produces no harsh impact on the musculoskeletal system. This happens as immersing in water reduces weight of our body. When we are immersed in water up to waist level, our weight is reduced by half. When immersed up to neck level, our weight is reduced by 90%. This means that when you are neck deep in water, you will be carrying only one tenth of your weight. This puts no strain on your body, however; you are still engaging in an intense workout. This is especially good to relieve joint and muscle aches as well as muscle stiffness. This is especially beneficial for those who are obese. In a few laps, swimming stretches, strengthens and provides aerobic exercise to the entire skeletal and muscular system. Even arthritic joints can be healed with a swim in warm water.

b. *It tones muscles and makes them stronger:* With every stroke in the pool, our body is pushing against water, which is twelve times denser than air. Swimming requires a dozen times more effort than walking! This in itself is a perfect resistance for muscles to build its strength and tone. With better muscles, the bones underneath it also get stimulated, which significantly reduces the chances of osteoporosis during old age.

c. *It improves the flexibility:* Swimming makes our joints and ligaments undergo a variety of movements in all directions, and makes them stay loose and flexible. Unlike working out in a gym where a single set of muscle is used, swimming moves the arms in circles, swings the hips and legs like a scissor, lengthens the body and twists the spine and head sideways. These efforts improve the balance and coordination of the whole body. Your baby could just become a tight-rope walker one day!

d. *It makes the heart and lungs healthier*: Swimming puts a tremendous demand on muscles, which increases their oxygen requirement. Heart starts beating stronger and faster to supply more oxygen. This puts demand on the lungs to supply oxygen and remove the carbon dioxide, which means breathing much deeper than regular. Over a period of years, heart and lungs become stronger and healthier. A healthier heart means more blood supply to all the organs. Swimmers are at very low risk of heart attack. A 30-minute daily dose of swimming reduces the chances of high-blood pressure and heart attack by 40%. Improved lung function is especially beneficial to children with asthma. Swimming from early childhood reduces the chances of severe asthmatic attacks. Furthermore, children with severe asthma also receive benefits due to increased lung volume done through swimming.

e. *It maintains a healthy weight:* Swimming is one of the fastest and easiest methods to burn calories. A short stint of 10-minutes can burn anywhere from 60 calories to up to 150 calories based on your body type and swimming style. A child regularly swimming into adulthood can never get obese!

f. *It keeps cholesterol at bay:* We have two types of cholesterols circulating and coordinating thousands of body functions in our body. The infamous bad (low-density cholesterol) cholesterol and highly desired good cholesterol (high-density cholesterol). To be healthy, a perfect ratio of concentration of these cholesterols needs to be maintained in the blood. For instance, with every one percent increase in high-density cholesterol, risk of death due to heart block is reduced by 3.5 percent. Swimming is a perfect aerobic exercise to get this ratio right by increasing concentration of high-density cholesterol. In addition, swimming maintains the strength and structure of arteries, thereby reducing deposition of cholesterol on its walls.

g. *It lowers the chances of diabetes:* aerobic exercise is one of the best proscriptions for reducing the chances of diabetes. For instance, with every 500 calories burnt, risk of acquiring type-2 diabetes is reduced by 10%. A breaststroke stint of just about half an hour in the pool burns more than 900 calories, reducing the chances of type-2 diabetes by 10%. In the case of diabetic patients, regular swimming increases insulin sensitivity, which is equivalent to the effects produced by anti-diabetic drugs.

h. *It boosts the efficiency of brain and lowers stress:* Regular swimmers are considered to be the happiest people. Swimming, through its overall health promoting benefits, makes you very happy. Happiness is just opposite of being sad, which comes with ailments. We feel happy when a group of neurotransmitters (brain chemicals) called endorphins are released. More endorphins more happiness! Whatever makes us happy, it does through stimulation of endorphin release.

The health benefits, and pleasant feelings association with swimming keeps the level of endorphins on a higher side. This is comparable to the effects of yoga, which also makes us happy. With happiness, stress is reduced, relaxation is achieved, and you will be ready to face any challenge. Furthermore, while swimming, we get disconnected from the outside world and noise, and are completely immersed in our movements, breathing and splash of water. Just like, we do during meditation! Swimming has been shown to have effects similar to meditation. During childhood, our brain cells grow and multiply in response to external stimulations. The multitudes of stimulating effects of swimming have the power to boost brain development. Also Swimming helps in the repair of damaged or degenerated neurons, which if left to heal naturally, may never recover!

i. *It Extends the lifespan:* With all the health benefits, swimming eventually extends your lifespan. In-fact, during these extended years you will not only be living, but you will be living a healthy and active life! Swimming is far ahead on this compared to other aerobic exercises. Long-term scientific studies have showed that swimming reduces the chances of death by 50 percent even when compared to walking or running.

C. It builds a strong bond between you and your baby

Numerous studies have proved that, skin to skin contact of mother and child immediately after birth and during initial months is one of the largest factors determining healthy growth and development. Newborns have no gut micro-flora and lacks body temperature maintaining abilities. A close contact with mother compensates for these two. Regular swimming means regular skin contact. These contacts strengthen the bond between the two. This is especially important for parents of more than one child. Swimming sessions can compensate for the loss of time to a child with short spans of intimate contacts.

D. It boosts confidence

Fear of water is one of the major hindrances in learning to swim at later stages in life. It is inherent.

We are born that way. This fear can grow in various ways we never recognise; like fear of sailing, fear of living near water-bodies, and so on. Exposing babies to swimming at early age prevents the development of fear later. Further, moving independently in water at early age also boosts confidence. Loaded with higher confidence levels, your baby can become a high achiever.

E. Swimming babies achieve better milestones

Early swimming builds mental and physical strengths that help in achieving all the milestones. Large-scale studies on Finnish children have proved that swimming babies start walking earlier than non-swimmers.

F. It develops their learning skills

Babies are exposed to instructive word repeatedly while swimming. For instance, they will hear kick, Kick, Hold on, side, turn, and so on in every training session. This exposure speeds up language learning and sharpens mental skills and level of understanding. For instance, it has been proved that swimming babies develop better motor as well as social skills, which is attributed to higher intelligence.

G. It makes babies easy to manage

Regular swimming sessions soothes and relaxes

your baby, and stimulates appetite and deep sleep. What else a mother can ask for!

H. **It is one of the best ways to have quality time**

Swimming sessions helps both parents as well as babies in spending time on meaningful and fun activities. At the same time developing and reaping the benefits. Swimming can be started from birth, even before your baby is vaccinated.

SWIMMING FOR BABIES

3. REASONS AND CRITERIA TO START EARLY

Swimming is not a sober activity. Swimming is fun for both adults and children. It is the best way to soothe your senses during vacation breaks. As we have seen in the previous section, swimming is one of the best forms of exercise with various amounts of benefits. It develops the body and the brain as well as building up endurance and stamina. It also protects the heart and lungs whilst it tones and tunes muscles and bones. Eventually, it adds healthy years to your life. Swimming is one of the very few wholesome lifetime exercises.

What more reasons are needed to stop your child from swimming?

Most people believe that swimming is not for children. Especially for children under the age of five. This is a myth. Swimming is especially good for children aged less than five years, and it can be started even from the day of birth. Yes, that is right, you can take your child to the pool even before the first-vaccination shot! Ideally, babies should be enrolled before the age of six. Babies have already done miles of swimming and bumping in the fluids of their mother's womb. It is just a matter of continuing this after birth.

Water phobia is one of the most common avoidable fears in men.

Water is part of human life. Swimming is a common activity at many community centres and gatherings for example camps, cruises and resorts. Water phobic people would be embarrassed in these gatherings. If the fear is serious and extends to waves, splashes and sprays, it will lead to life-limiting effects. Furthermore, fear of water can extend if unresolved early to fear of bathing (ablutophobia). This rare manifestation can be devastating. For instance, it would lower the hygiene standards, leading to regular serious infections.

Teaching swimming at early ages is the best method to avoid water phobia. Infants can have both negative as well as positive reactions to new exposures. The positive responses can be channelled to embrace swimming and altogether prevent the chances of aquaphobia. A lifelong wonderful journey with water is what your child will get.

Coming to the best time to start swimming, a lot of confusion exists as different coaching centres have their own standards. Six months is a scientifically suitable time for starting swimming classes. At this age, your child would have developed stronger muscles and bones, which could withstand the pressure of water. This is also the right age for babies to accept newer experiences through physical involvement. If not standing, most of the six-month olds would have learnt sitting and crawling, which would help in learning swimming.

Some schools suggest starting babies from three months of age by initiating simple leg and arm movements in a bathtub. This will prepare the baby to learn to swim easily at six months.

However, it completely depends on you to decide the best time to enrol your baby for swimming classes. Each baby is unique. Some babies are fast learners and others are not; some grow faster and others slower; some fear water and other enjoy. Among these factors, the most important is a well developed body structure. If a four month old has developed a strong bone and muscles system, he is ready to swim. On the contrary, a ten month old may not be suitable for swimming if he has week bones or muscle.

Twins William and Ellenita Trykush, created a splash by swimming the length of a 25-metre pool at just nine months old, and fifteen-months-old Maharanth had already mastered the ability to swim four meters underwater! These children were guided by a paediatrician and certified coaches. Hence, it is advisable to consult a paediatrician and a certified swimming trainer who will be able to guide on all the aspects of swimming. One rule of thumb for deciding is to check whether your baby is already sitting, crawling and trying to stand on their own. If the answer to all of these is yes, your baby will be better able to balance, which will help in withstanding the pressure of water.

Another important criterion is the health and immunity of your baby. In case he is prone to frequent bouts of infections, asthma attacks or is carrying a birth defect, only a paediatrician can be able to decide on enrolling him for swimming.

You need to remember that when a baby is exposed to too much water, some of them will react negatively. This is something a parent should try to avoid to prevent illnesses and complications. Even a healthy baby can become ill on exposure to water due to negative attitudes. Watch carefully to understand the reactions of your baby to water on first-pool exposure.

Finally, your swimming abilities do play a big role in your child's learning curve. If you are an expert swimmer, you will be able to teach the baby faster with your confidence. So, take the plunge first, and you will be able to enjoy the benefits of swimming together with your baby. Your home cannot be a replacement for well equipped swimming schools as these schools will have trained coaches and will be able to handle the situation better in case of emergencies.

4. INFLUENCE OF PARENTS ON YOUR BABY'S SWIMMING SKILLS

To a large extent, a child becomes what his parents make of him. For instance, studies have proved that authoritative parenting increases the social and emotional skills of children. These children learn judgement skills early and go on to become better individuals. To develop a confident and authoritative nature, you need to be skilled and have control over your behaviour. Yes, I mean to say that you should be able to swim and be confident around water if you are expecting your child to learn to swim quickly.

Attitudes of children towards water starts shaping from the first time he is bathed. Parent's behaviour during bathing shapes baby's perceptions of water. This influences the baby's learning speed during the actual exposure to swimming pool later. Hence, parents should be aware of their verbal and physical cues during bathing. Either, positive or negative emotions will be passed on to the child with equal chances. So, you should be careful if you are not comfortable around water. For instance, when your baby goes near the water, and if you react by grabbing quickly and pulling with loud verbal suggestion that "water can be dangerous and should be avoided," it will instil negative feelings in the baby about water. With time and after some repetitions, this feeling will become stronger. This will prolong the time required for your baby to embrace water during swimming lessons.

On first-introduction and initial exposure of babies to the pool, parents should exude positive enthusiasm. Parents are the world for babies, and all the responses of the father or mother to any external stimuli will be adopted by babies. Hence, parents need to be positive and relaxed from beginning to the end of every swimming session.

A parent's body language is an important component of ensuring early swim lessons go smoothly, and is integral to the success of the water familiarization and learn-to-swim processes. A parent who is nervous and clings to their child or holds them out of the water sends a message to the child is in an unsafe environment. Instead, the parent in the swim lesson should remain relaxed with your shoulders at the water's surface or just below, and gently support the child in the water, or alternatively, if the child is old enough, they should encourage the independence of the baby in the water and allow the baby to hold on to them. Parent's attitudes become the single largest factor if you are training your baby on your own, either at the pool or at home.

You can make full benefit from the coaching classes through listening to and understanding all the instructions, by asking questions specifically important for your child, and active participation in activities and discussions. And obviously, you should be ready to get wet every-time with full enthusiasm. However, if you do not know swimming, you may be subtly expressing your negative feelings like fear towards water. Do try to keep these at minimal, to help your child gain confidence in swimming. Most of the swimming schools do not need parent's active participation, but your participation can boost the confidence of your child and hasten the learning process. This way, you will be letting the child know that it is not harmful to get into the water.

In many schools, instructors take help of parents to facilitate teaching. Parents know their child better than anybody else. Children react to parent's praises better than other words. Parents can use this to positively reinforce learning through regular praise at each and every opportunity, starting from entering into the pool to learning to swim. Praise every new skill, however minor it may seem. On the other side, always be careful not to fall into the comparison trap. Every child has its own pace of learning that is mostly determined genetically through parents. Never compare your child with other fast learning children. Always remember that you have taken your child to swimming pool to teach him swimming, but not to humiliate him with comparison. Comparison will lead the activity to lose its sense of fun.

The role of parent in child learning is one of the most ignored factors. It is vital for a parent to be there and show the way for a child to learn to swim through demonstrations, especially if your child is less than four years. Along with helping your child to learn how to swim, it will also strengthen the bond between you and your child.

5. THINGS TO BUY BEFORE STARTING

Swimming lessons are a perfect exercise for any child, and are especially necessary if you are living near water bodies. Well, you have thought-it-over and decided to enrol your child in a swimming school. The date for first lesson is near and you will start wondering whether you have everything you need to pack for the classes. Well, here is a checklist, of essentials as well as optional, which you can improve upon based on your child's specific requirements.

Before buying a list, grab a waterproof backpack to carry your child's belongings. Think of all the things he needs at a time. Like an extra pair of clothes, a set of swim diapers, towels, swimwear, and pull-up if your baby is still not potty trained. Most of the swim schools require your baby to be bathed before and after swimming. A bar of soap in a waterproof case will be useful to bath with. In case the swimming school is outdoors, an insect spray and sunscreen lotion will be very helpful. Include an additional plastic bag to carry the wet clothes and towels back home after the classes.

Your full work and home contact details as well as mobile phone numbers must be provided to the designated instructor in order to facilitate immediate contact in case of an emergency. If possible, contacts of both the parents will be more helpful. Further, the instructor can be authorised to take medical decisions in case they fail to contact you during medical emergencies. A bag with a list of allergies, medications, dose and schedule should be included in the bag or should be handed over to the designated instructor.

Thousands of varieties of swimming toys are available on the market to choose from. You can decide based on the directions of the instructor, as they will have specific guidelines for allowing toys. One or two of your baby's favourite toys should be enough. Swimming goggles are usually not recommended for children as they hamper vision and may delay learning. However, if your child is using contact lenses, goggles will be an essential item. Similarly, nose or ear plugs are advised only if specifically required.

After the swim class, your child will be quite hungry; a small pack of snack and drink will be very useful. Follow the school guidelines for food in class.

This list is not exhaustive. It may also seem to be a big task for some. Remember that baby swim classes hardly last more than an hour. Pack accordingly. Minimal and essentials will do the job.

Do not go overboard, as your child is not going to college!

6. BEST PRACTICES FOR BABY SWIMMING CLASSES

We tend to expect a lot from our children. We buy all the best stuff and enrol the child in the best of swimming schools in town. Now, it is the child's turn to do his part and learn the swimming with ease. This is a natural but completely wrong approach to teaching swimming to babies. The child learns to swim at his own pace. Our expectations and pressure are only going to slow down his pace. Net outcome will be disappointment after a few classes. To prevent such an episode we can consciously follow some guidelines and achieve better results:

1. *Appreciate that your child is unique:* Every child has his own ways and speeds of learning. Your child may be fast at swimming and slow at other things, or vice-versa. Appreciate him for this. In case he is not at all able to learn even after prolonged teaching. Have a critical look at the teaching style. The methods may not be suitable for him. Try to use a different method

altogether. Find the right method for him. Some children learn by observing others whereas others like to learn by practice.

2. *Acknowledge every achievement:* Every small step, from getting into the pool for the first time to his first stroke, however small it may seem, it is a big stride in the learning process of the child. Appreciate this. Acknowledge these milestones without fail. It will make him confident! No big things are needed to achieve this; a big smile and a lovely hug will do the job. Tell him he is doing great, he will understand.

3. *Comfort first:* Make sure your baby is comfortable in the water before starting the first lesson. At first, the child could be highly uncomfortable in the water. Keep him relaxed. The idea is to take his mind away from the pool to make him stay in the pool for a few minutes. Tell him short stories or sing to him to make him forget that he is in the water. Assure him that you are holding him, and he is safe. A few of these efforts will comfort him. Tell him about other children having fun in the water and ask him to follow them. The earlier he gets comfortable in the water, the faster will be his learning.

4. *Socialise your baby:* Swimming classes are a social activity. Introduce your baby to other children and their parents. In a few days, he will have made a few good friends, whom he will like to follow. If possible, make them learn together. It will double the fun and speedup the learning process. Babies always look for fun. Exploit this to impart learning. And you never know a minor competition may be sparked with a friend, which is good for both. However, do not let this competition go overboard. Keep it healthy.

5. *Involve family members in swimming:* As many times possible, include family members in swimming lessons and demonstrations. This will make learning a fun activity. This will also strengthen the bond of all the members with your baby. And, your skills will also be honed.

6. *Learning by seeing precedes learning by doing:* Be attentive and professional all the time. Learn all the instructions and follow. Be a great role model. You will be the first-role model your child likes to follow, eventhough he has an instructor. Your child will be looking at you for cues and directions. Be

conscious of this. Babies will try to learn by seeing initially, but they can only learn best by doing. Be organized, disciplined and honest. Perform the swimming steps before your baby. Let him see you and learn.

7. *Do not hinder learning:* Inability of children to satisfy the expectations of parents can lead to regular bursts of disappointments. Children are very sensitive to the expressions of parents. They can sense this. This can hinder their learning process. Exactly opposite of what your encouragement can do. Follow a simple principal to avoid this situation. Get into the shoes of your child and minimise the expectations to a reasonable level. After-all he is just a child.

8. *Teach your child one-step at a time:* As adults, even if we are horrible at swimming, we have at-least seen many swimming pools and understand the meaning of swimming. We may learn fast and even jump some steps. This cannot be expected from a child to whom the swimming pool is a completely alien world. But he will learn eventually. Let him learn a single step at a time. Let him master it and then take him to the next step. It is also essential to gauging whether he is mentally and physically ready to learn new

steps.

9. *Maintain your calm:* The speed of your baby's learning may frustrate you, especially if you are short tempered. Hold on. Do not break the ceiling. Also maintain your temper when baby indulges in bad habits like swallowing the water. If your baby sees you repeatedly losing temper, he may eventually get scared of water and lose interest in swimming. And then, it will be very difficult to start again. Just go with his pace and mischief.

Your baby should always trust you: Completely avoid wrong practices like lying or unexpected acts like throwing him suddenly into the water. Prepare him well before every act. Maintain his trust. He will repay your trust by learning what you teach.

7. TEACHING BABIES TO SWIM

a. Infants

As discussed above, newborns have been through swimming and know the basics. Teaching swimming to an infant is not a simple task. It involves a lot of carefully planned and executed steps. Before going through the actual methods, you have to plan well the following: the swimming atmosphere, location, time of the day, feeding and the method of swimming. Keep the swimming area organized and clean. Create a schedule and maintain a similar time of the day for swimming lessons.

Babies should be well fed before swimming. Avoid taking both hungry as well as just-fed babies into the water. Use the same location or tub for swimming lessons to minimize distractions. The methods should be followed inorder starting with simple to complex. Follow these simple steps to ensure that your infant learns how to swim quickly. The methods listed below are suitable for three-month-old babies.

Start with a hug and cuddle

Hug your baby and cuddle him, whenever you reach him towards the water. This reassures your baby of safety. You can recline in the water with your baby face to face with you; continuously looking into each other's eyes. Water level should be up to your chest level. Allow your baby to lie on you, face to face. All the times, taking care to keep his head from dipping. Repeat this activity for few days, and he will start efforts to stand on his legs. Let him stand, initially for a few seconds and your full support. Some efforts later, he will start standing for a longer time and in a straighter position. This will give him the strength required to kick into the water.

Teach him the balancing

Slowly, when he is fully comfortable, start to let go of him for a brief time after the initial cuddle in the reclined position, for about one to two seconds. Make sure that your baby is not sliding into the water; gently steadying him before his chin reaches water level. This will teach your baby balancing skills in water. Repeat this for subsequent days. Taking sides and making minor changes every time. You will find that within a week, your child will be able to reposition and hold on to you from either left or right sides. With this your baby will be able to learn balancing and floating.

Teach him to float on the back

As you sit in the tub and turn him around to bring his chest up, your child may get nervous as he loses eye contact with you. Your baby will be frightened at this stage. Comfort him with gentle words and soft repeated touches. After a short time bring him back and make eye contact. After a few days, he will be comfortable lying on his back. With your free hand start lifting him at his back, so that his lower body can float. Now, one of your hands is supporting his head and neck, and another should be holding the buttocks.

Repeat this for many days and he will get comfortable and starts enjoying and kicking in this position. At this stage, if you slowly start leaving him and re-holding him just after he comes down one or two inches, he will eventually start floating on his back. Some babies may take a very longer time to achieve this. The trick is to maintain both the body and mind relaxed. A tensed baby will become denser and drown faster.

Teaching to blow water out and hold the breath in

With your baby face to face and watching you, lower yourself up to chin in the tub. Show that you are very excited about what you are going to do next by laughing and giggling loudly.Now start blowing bubbles towards him. Let him see it. He will love it and enjoy it. Your baby will also start imitating the blowing action that you are doing. Let him blow, making sure to keep his nose above water level. In case he tries gulping water, guide him repeatedly. This will teach him to avoid drinking water during swimming.

Babies instantly close eyes if you blow air on their faces. With the closed eyes, the baby also holds its breath for a few seconds. This can be used to teach your baby to hold breath underwater. Gently blow a breath and dip him under water as he closes the eyes, and bring back slowly and steadily before he starts inhaling. This simple exercise will teach your baby the art of holding breath during a dive.

Teaching to go up and down

Hold your baby beneath armpits face-to-face chin deep in water. Lift him straight up as much as possible, and bring him back to chin-deep position. Babies love this exercise. Keep the temperature of air and water closer. Water will be splashing on baby's face during the dip, prompting him to close the eyes and hold the breath. When he is comfortable with this exercise, allow him to get into the water whilst you hold and lift him. This will teach him getting into the water and coming out with holding breath and preventing water entering into the mouth. The baby may gulp water many times. Allow him to cough it out and restart after a break.

This exercise should be done in stages with initially dipping him up to chin, and then up to the mouth, and then nose and followed by up to eyes and finally to a full submersion. Also, make sure to pull him up before he gulps or inhales water when submersed. Eventually, the baby will learn to hold breath underwater for few seconds. This is the single major factor that influences swimming learning process. The breath holding can be programmed with a rhyme or counting from 1 to 4 or whatever verbal signal that your baby likes. Repeating the submersion and lifting process with the verbal gesture will ingrain the steps into baby's brain. Alternatively, holding baby under shower can be used to teach breath holding.

Eventually, with few months of these sessions, your baby will also accomplish sitting into the tub and holding on sides firmly. He may also learn to stand up firmly holding your hands. Be consistent and regular during these periods. Now, your baby can be taken face down into the water for a moment, and he will start holding breath and enjoying the kicks. He will start floating with some practice, but only for a few seconds.

b. Six months to one year

As the lessons progress, the home tub or baby pool will become smaller for your infant. At this stage, a smooth transition should be made to a bigger pool. Babies can swim in the bathtub up to six to nine months of age based on their growth. During the transition, initial stages should involve just exposure to the new pool with continued activity in the old tub. Slowly increasing time from the older to the newer pool till complete transition is done. For instance, if your baby were swimming daily for half an hour, perhaps five minutes of this could be shifted to a new setting. This should be preferably sandwiched between times at the regular pool. Gradually increase the five minutes to full time.

A typical concern with the transition to public pools is temperature and hygiene. Unlike the home atmosphere, where the temperature can be easily maintained. Such control is not guaranteed at most of the public pools or schools. Similarly, it becomes your responsibility to ensure that proper hygiene and baby safe chemicals are used for the maintenance of pools. It is advisable to have a detailed consultation with a trainer as well as a paediatrician during this transition.

Your baby can continue the similar breath

holding, bogging and floating exercises in the new pool. Do not immediately start teaching new steps. Instead, focus on giving him an opportunity to explore the new pool gradually allowing longer durations of classes. This should increase his breath-holding abilities and duration. With these classes, by the age of one year, your baby should be able to hold the breath longer, sit on the side of the pool, swim underwater (feet or two), jump into and come to the surface to take a breath. Most important, he should be able to do these with minimal or no assistance. This can be achieved through a set of six activities he is already familiar with:

1. *Snuggling*: Snug, hug, praise and cuddle your baby as much as possible with every opportunity. Snuggle to praise new accomplishment. Snuggle to give him a break. And snuggle for everything else!

2. *Floating face up*: Floating on the back can be continued exactly like earlier. Floating can be a lesson as well as a rest between lessons. Make sure to increase the un-holding time, such that he may start floating independently at the age of one year! Remember, floating is all about a relaxed mind and body.

3. *Submersion*: This is the most important

lesson. Use the verbal cue for which your baby was adapted to submersion and practice gentle submersion by allowing him to go down in a horizontal position and snuggle with praises after he comes up. Slowly, add movements along with submersion. When he is a few inches underwater, make him move gently between two objects or persons placed about 2 meters apart. The distance can be gradually increased parallel to his breath holding ability.

At this stage, you can also include jumping in lessons by seating him on the edge of the pool. Standing in the water, using a verbal cue like 1-2-3, make him jump into the water and get him out after a very brief period. After some repetitions, he will be able to do it without your assistance. He will also start jumping with a higher force and swim up farther. Give him more room. Exactly opposite to it, your baby can easily learn to climb out of the pool with your assistance. Instead of seating him for jumping, make him try himself to climb out with you gently pushing him from the bottom. His eagerness to take the next jump will make him learn climbing out very quickly.

4. *Bubble blowing:* Like earlier stages, continue the bubble blowing lessons. At this stage, a

whistle can be used to blow the bubbles with different sounds. It makes it much more interesting and fun. It will increase his breath-holding duration.

5. *Bobbing*: Similarly, continue bobbing up and down, gradually increasing the underwater time as his breath-holding capacity improves.

6. *End with a Play*: At the end of the lessons, start including short, playful activities that are not in order of the lessons. These playful activities can encourage multiple skills at a time as they are integrated together with the lessons. Increase the duration of play gradually. Always keep them at the end, or else your baby will be exhausted to learn other lessons!

c. One year to three years

As your baby celebrates his first birthday, he would have learnt the lessons from previous two sections. His coaching can now continue to the next level. Your baby can be now called a swimmer, and from now on the swimming classes will have tremendous influence over his growth and development.

To recapitulate, the principals learnt during previous stages should be maintained. Keep the snuggling on, maintain the regularity, and follow the schedule diligently. At the end of three years, your child should be proficient in diving into the pool, swimming a 6 yards width, and climbing out independently. However, it should not be allowed in your absence. The thumb rule is to lift him before he inhales and stop him before he is fatigued! Further, increase the length of the lessons gradually to get him adapted.

Following is a general list of activities that you can teach your baby during one to three years of age. You are free to improvise!

1. *Holding on to the sides of the pool:* Position yourself with child holding on to the sides. Let him hold independently. Do this during every lesson and increase gradually. This

will help him when taking breaks or climbing out of the pool faster in case of emergencies.

2. *Thrusting off the side:* Standing on to the sides, teach him to push off into the water. From a few inches at first to few meters. You can stand in the pool and invite him after he has learnt the technique. Every time increasing the distance.

3. *Approaching the steps of the pool:* Standing at a short distance from the steps, make your child swim towards the steps still holding onto him. Repeat plenty of times. He will love the site of approaching steps gradually. Increase the distance with every few sessions.

4. *Improved floating on the back:* He is already doing it from previous sessions! Just increase the time and make him move gently.

5. *Swimming from the steps:* After your baby has mastered swimming towards steps, initiate him to learn to swim away from the steps. Put your baby on the steps with him half submerged in water (up to chest level). Holding his hands gently, ask him to swim towards you. As he improves, increase the

distance gradually and make him swim without your assistance.

6. *Swimming in a current:* Holding your baby under armpits in a horizontal position, create a current with body movements and gently leave him and step back. Asking him to swim at you. This will simulate the conditions from a stream, beach or the water movements of a public pool. Increase the distance and intensity of the water current.

7. *Getting out of the pool:* Climbing out of the pool can be taught at either side or through the steps. Assist him in climbing out and then reduce the assistance gradually to make him independent.

8. *Using the ladder:* Learning to climb out of the steps may not be enough. Many of the pools have ladders in place of steps. Standing close to the ladder assist him in climbing out like you did for steps. He should learn it rapidly as the side rails will help him. Similarly, teach him stepping down and jumping from the ladder.

9. *Swim-surface-swim:* Holding under his armpits in a horizontal position, release him

in the water and step back slowly. Ask him to swim towards you. As required help him to come to surface and then repeat the earlier steps. Repeat this, every time reducing the level of assistance. This will teach him to surface and swim independently.

10. *Jumping and diving:* Keep your child on the side, make him hold your finger and ask him to jump. Gradually allow him to do it independently. Couple this with increasing distance and his jump should improve. Similarly, he can be trained to dive, first from kneeling position and then standing at the edge. He should be guided to master shallow dive and forward movement, not a deep dive! Diving from the standing position needs much more care as water should not be shallow. It is better to keep diving from standing position as the last lesson towards third year of his age.

d. Three years to six years

By three years, your child must have mastered jumping in the water, swimming about six meters and climb out independently. One specialty of three-year olds is that they are highly active and can get very excited. Keep them well fed and nourished. Swimming takes a lot of their energy.

At the age of three years, your baby can be initiated to learn a complete stroke involving multiple steps. However, during training the individual steps should be taught separately. Once he has mastered all the steps, they can be combined to make the complete stroke. As an example, he can be taught the famous crawl stroke as follows:

1. *Learning to breathe properly:* Your child should now learn to co-ordinate inhaling and exhaling with swimming movements. Many different methods are followed for this. One of the simplest is by standing on the edge with both the hands holding on to the sides, with the face into the water, make him to touch chin to the left shoulder and inhale. Follow this with the return of the chin to its position and exhale. Alternate sides can be used to learn this technique.

2. *Learning to use the arms:* This step involves teaching your child to pick an arm out of the water, extending it over the head, putting it back into the water and pulling it through. Standing in shallow water, hold the child at your hip level on the water with one hand, with another hand lift his hand on the other side, extend, put it back and make a pulling movement. Keep his fingers close together. It can be repeated eight times for each hand. Your child will learn to do it on his own.

3. *Learning to flutter kick the legs:* Flutter kick involves moving the whole leg from the hip, keeping the knees straight. This helps in keeping the body horizontal and propel forward. Holding on to the sides, it can be taught similar to using the arms, beginning with about eight kicks for each session. You will be holding the baby with one hand under his chest, and another under his thighs.

4. *Streamlining:* This step involves learning to keep the body straight. Streamlining helps in easy forward movements. Assist him to keep the arms straight ahead, one on another, with the body maintained straight from the fingertips to the feet. This step is complicated

and will take a significant amount of time. Once he learns it, ask him to jump from the side and swim towards you in a streamlined stroke!

After your child has mastered the four steps individually, his brain is ready to combine them as required. For instance, you can teach him to combine breathing and kicking, or breathing-kicking-use of arms. Include playtime at the end!

At the end of five years, your child should be able to swim 12 meters of the pool with crawl stroke. You can swim along to make it interesting!

Starting from around four to five years, based on when he learns to do the crawl stroke independently, your focus should be shifted from teaching new skills to improving the existing skills. He has learnt a great deal. It is time to make him perfect. This can be done by improving the quality of streamlining, improving endurance, improving the stroke quality and finally mastering the dive. Repeated and regular sessions of combinations of crawl strokes will be enough to achieve these benefits.

8. WATER SAFETY AND HYGIENE

Poor water hygiene and safety provisions can run your child into serious injuries or acute infections. Here is a guideline on determining if the swimming pool you are looking at is good for you.

The Center of Disease Control (CDC) and the World Health Organization (WHO) have set forth the following recommendations to consider before entering into a swimming pool:

1. Avoid taking children with any illness, especially diarrhoea into the pool. He can spread the disease to others.

2. Teach your child not to drink or gulp water from the pool.

3. Hygiene should be the priority. Shower your child before getting into the pool and after coming out of the pool.

4. Keep a watch on the diaper and take children to washrooms from urinal. Use swimming diapers in babies not trained for potty. Wash your child with soap when changing diaper.

5. Use ear plugs in case your child has an ear infection.

Following precautions will further ensure the health and safety of your child at the pool:

1. Children should be continuously under the supervision of parents or trainers at least till they reach ten years of age.
2. Children below three years of age must be kept away from older children or adult pools. Separate pools should be provided for these children.
3. Crowded swimming pools should be avoided.
4. Swimming is not only a fun exercise; it is a life saving skill.
5. At home, prevent access to a swimming pool in your absence. Do not keep your baby's toys near the edges of the pool.
6. Babies should not be allowed to run alongside the pool. They may slip and fall dangerously.
7. Special plastic shoes with grips can be used to avoid slipping.
8. Use hand floaters and life jacket generously, till your baby can swim independently.

Practice those tips and enjoy the summer with your kids.

9. AUTHOR'S NOTE

Dear reader,

Thank you very much for reading this book. Teaching your child to swim is an exciting and meaningful journey for both of you. I will be very happy when I receive great feedback from you on reading and learning from this book. I hope you liked this book as much as I enjoyed writing it.

To read more articles that are interesting and to download a video training course on baby swimming, visit our website by following the QR code below. Just scan it with your Smartphone QR code reader and it will take you to the page.

Your feedback is very important to me. If you enjoyed reading this book and you have a few minutes to spare, may I ask that, you leave a great review on Amazon. Even a short review is fine. Reviews help me spread the word about the book and encourage me to keep writing.

Thank you again.

Kind regards,
Mark Dube

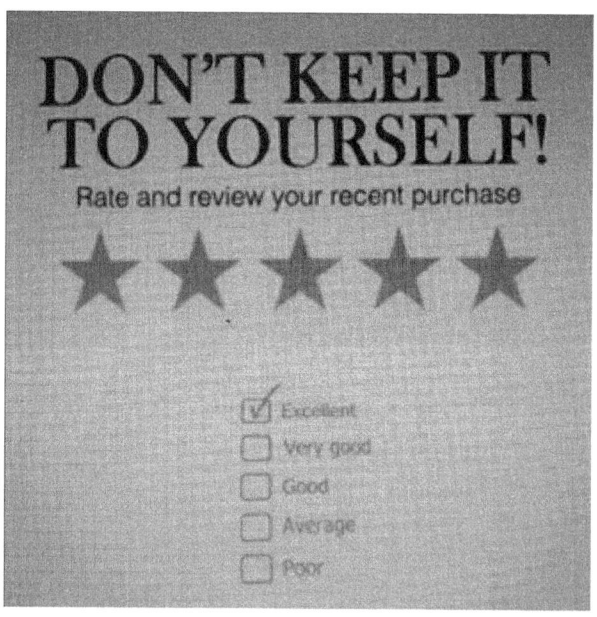